MW01600471

Understanding Infertility

Insights for Family and Friends

by

Patricia Irwin Johnston

Perspectives Press
P.O. Box 90318
Indianapolis IN 46290-0318

This book is dedicated to the thousands of fertility-impaired people—my peers—whom it has been my honor to meet and correspond with and provide workshops for and work alongside during an adult lifetime spent first as a volunteer and later as a professional in the fields of infertility and family building alternatives. May their struggle be more respected by those whose lives touch theirs.

Toward Understanding!
PIJ
August, 1996

Other in-print books by Pat Johnston...

Perspectives on a Grafted Tree
Taking Charge of Infertility
Adopting after Infertility
Launching a Baby's Adoption

This booklet has been adapted and revised from the 1983 booklet *Understanding: A Guide to Impaired Fertility for Family and Friends*.

Y ou are reading this booklet because someone you know—a co-worker, perhaps, or a neighbor, or a member of your family or a close friend—is experiencing a problem in trying to start or expand a family. They find themselves infertile. This person or couple needs your support at this time as they would during any other life crisis. However, those who have not themselves experienced infertility may find it especially hard to offer help which an infertile person seems to be able to feel is appropriate. Even friends or family members who themselves dealt with infertility before the mid-1980s and so assume they "know what it's like," experienced something very different from what today's infertile couples go through.

Up to now you may not have thought much about infertility at all. You may have conceived easily yourself—in fact you may have conceived without wanting to! In high school sex ed classes they warned us to stay out of the back seats of cars, they lectured about untimely pregnancies, they cautioned us about venereal diseases, but they didn't tell us anything about the one in six couples who will experience a fertility impairment. As a result, on first hearing about your friends' problem, you may have tried to comfort them by blurting out something like,

"Relax, maybe you're trying too hard. Why don't you have a glass of wine before bedtime (or take a vacation, or light a few candles, or hang a maternity dress in the closet)"... or

"You've got plenty of time! Really, You don't know how great you've got it with two incomes and no kids!"... or

"I don't know, it seems to be in the water around here. All Charlie has to do is look at me!"... or

"You know, I know you're seeing some big time reproductive endocrinologist in the city, but my friend Shirley's sister was having trouble getting pregnant, and then she saw this doc (or nutritionist or acupuncturist, etc.) over in Smallville and she got pregnant right away."...or

"You really think you want kids, huh? Here, take my three-year-old why don'tcha?"

And what happened when you made something like one of these meant-to-be-supportive statements to your infertile friend? I'd be willing to bet that it was met with stony silence or a forced smile or a dropped jaw or perhaps even a sudden teary exit. This booklet is designed to offer you some basic education so that you can understand impaired fertility more fully and respond accordingly.

THE PROBLEM

What is infertility? Infertility is most commonly defined as the inability to conceive after a year of unprotected intercourse, but it also describes the inability to carry a pregnancy to a live birth. This definition includes a variety of situations. For example, people who have been trying to have a baby for a year but haven't gotten pregnant are infertile, but so are people who have become pregnant but have miscarried several times, and so, too are people who have successfully given birth before but who are not able to do so again when they want to.

While pregnancy occurs in a female's body, the absence of a pregnancy is not necessarily a symptom of a problem with her reproductive system. About half of couples who have trouble conceiving discover that the problem causing the infertility is in the male partner's body. The statistics say that 30-40% of couples find female fertility impairments, another 30-40% discover male fertility problems, another 30% or so find that both partners' reproductive systems have a problem. In fewer than 10% of cases (and this number is shrinking every year) modern medicine just can't identify a specific problem that is causing the fertility impairment.

The good news for infertile couples is that, with appropriate medical care (note that term, *appropriate*), almost 70% of them can be helped to become pregnant and deliver a child who is genetically related to them both. Furthermore, the proportion of couples who can and will become pregnant is also increasing steadily. This is hardly ever easy, however, and we are going to discuss later how you can be supportive of what may prove to be a long and difficult and expensive and distressing and painful treatment process.

Well over half of couples who experience impaired fertility will face a long term challenge. Even those couples who eventually conceive and give birth to a child genetically related to both of them will very likely have spent some time exploring (quite privately for the most part) several alternatives to continued medical treatment. Many couples will eventually decide to pursue one or more of these alternatives.

Some will consider whether to collaborate with a third party—a donor—whose reproductive abilities are not impaired in order to make a

4

baby. Sometimes these options involving collaborative reproduction are called gamete adoptions, because they very often result in a couple parenting a child who is genetically related to one of the parents who raise him, but not to the other, who, in essence, "adopts" him. For example, if the medical problem is male infertility, one alternative is using sperm from another man for the wife to conceive. This is called donor insemination, and most often involves an unknown donor, though sometimes a family member or friend agrees to donate his sperm. When the problem is with some part of the wife's reproductive system, there are several third party alternatives. For quite some time now surrogates have been willing to be inseminated with the sperm of a man whose wife is infertile and to give birth to a baby genetically related to the surrogate and the husband of the infertile woman. In these cases the wife then legally adopts her husband's child. But now there are additional alternatives involving third party reproductive assistance for women. A couple may use donated ova (eggs) fertilized with the husband's sperm in vitro (outside the body) and then have the resulting embryo transferred to the wife's uterus so that she will experience a pregnancy and give birth to the baby even though she is not genetically related to it. Other infertile women may have eggs but not be able to sustain a pregnancy. For these couples, using a surrogate to carry and give birth to a baby which has been conceived in vitro using the husband's sperm and the wife's ova may be the best answer. In a few cases both donated eggs and donated sperm are used. Using collaborative, third party assisted reproductive options it is medically, technically, and legally possible—though not at all common—for a child to have three sets of parents: an infertile couple who arrange for the conception of a child they will eventually adopt and parent; genetic parents who donate their sperm and ova (and who are unlikely to be married to one another); a genetically-unrelated surrogate who carries the resulting pregnancy to term and her husband, who, under most existing laws, would be the legal father of any child to whom his wife gives birth until the two of them transfer their parental rights to the infertile couple for adoption.

Other couples will explore more traditional adoption as an option. In fact, this is the option that is most commonly "recommended" to infertile couples by well-meaning but too often misinformed others. Adoption, which has been around for a very long time, has changed a great deal in the last decade and a half. There are far fewer newborns available for adoption (primarily because single parenthood is no longer stigmatized) but many more older children with very special needs. Adopting couples now have many choices to make. Should they adopt a baby or an older child (or even a sibling group)? Should they adopt through an agency or try on their own to find a birthmother and arrange what's called a private adoption? Could they consider adopting a child who is racially or ethnically different from themselves? Would it be best for them to explore adoption only here at home, or should they consider international adoption? Would they be comfortable with openness in the relationship with their child-to-be's birthfamily, or would they prefer a completely confidential adoption?

Still other couples will look carefully at their treatment options and at the collaborative family-building alternatives and at adoption and will decide that their lives really can be full and productive without their experiencing parenthood after all, and so, after much soul searching and careful deliberation, they will choose to see themselves no longer as child<u>less</u>, but instead as child<u>free</u>.

We'll spend more time talking about these options later, but if this all sounds too complicated for comfort already, you are beginning to have some idea of why infertility is so difficult for couples to experience! In fact, if reading just these few paragraphs has been enough to make you want to toss up your hands and find something else to do, the rest of this booklet is <u>exactly</u> what your infertile friends need for you to concentrate on for the next hour or so.

THE BACKGROUND

Those born from the mid-1940s to the early 1960s—the generation who are referred to as the Baby Boomers—were part of the first generation in history to come to adulthood expecting to be in control of their reproductive lives. Earlier generations had relied upon abstinence, inconsistently effective barrier methods, and calendar counting known as "rhythm" in their attempts to control fertility. But the Boomers had ready, reliable, inexpensive access to The Pill, which produced a kind of reproductive freedom with which their parents and grandparents couldn't even identify! The ready availability of reliable birth control resulted in a "sexual revolution" which produced, among many other things, new attitudes about age at marriage and for family formation, number of sexual partners, etc. Now, a generation and a half after The Pill's development during the 1950s and '60s, <u>everything</u> about fertility and infertility has changed more than it had during any other span of time in western culture.

The result?... There has never been a better time or a worse time to be infertile than now, at the dawn of the 21st century.

On the one hand, rapid advancements in technology, in drug research and in surgery which bring new ideas and new treatments in frequent and rapid succession offer tremendous hope to infertile couples. Specialized help in the form of microsurgical and laser surgical experts, hormone specialists, in vitro fertilization clinics, etc., are available in virtually every large city and major medical center and even in many middle sized cities. The result is that truly expert help is available within a few hours drive of even the most isolated rural communities of the United States.

On the other hand, though there's more information about infertility available today than ever before, there seems to be less compassion for the infertile. Society encourages the careful planning of lives to include education, training, and carefully established careers with financial security before parenthood begins. We are encouraged to eat healthily, to play healthily, to be active and fit. Many, if not most couples, then, spend large parts of their potentially fertile years trying diligently <u>not</u> to become pregnant, presuming in this age of good health and controllable fertility that if and when they do wish to have a baby they will do so easily.

One would expect that in an era touting Family Values—a backlash reaction to the troublesome side effects of the '60s' sexual revolution—there would be compassion for the infertile. In an age where hospital marketing departments compete with one another to promote their pregnancy and delivery-related services of exercise and nutrition classes, child-birth preparation, birthing rooms and chairs and pools as <u>the</u> key to good bonding with baby-to-be, one would expect some understanding and support for those who want a baby but can't seem to make one. But too many fertile people have little patience for the infertile and what they see as "obsessive" attempts to become pregnant.

The misunderstood promise of fertility control has prompted increasing numbers of couples to delay parenthood to their naturally less fertile 30s and even moreso into their 40s and 50s, complicating attempts at pregnancy. The ever-lengthening menu of treatment options has substantially blurred the view of a clear stopping point. And as a society obsessed as well with population control, we don't seem to care.

Here's a personal view... My husband and I are a second generation infertile couple. Dave's parents dealt with infertility during the 1930s and '40s, losing several babies they had conceived together and ultimately building their family by adoption. Dave and I married in the '60s and began our marriage feeling very powerful about our fertility. We would go on The Pill until I graduated from college and then—unlike my own parents, who had had three children in diapers at the same time—we would space our children exactly three years apart.

For Dave's parents and other infertile people of the generation before our own there was little help and therefore little hope. Because there were few treatments available, answers about how far to go were relatively clear. But then, in general people had lower expectations about what medical treatment of any kind could do for them. Accepting "what came along" was a cultural given before World War II. Because the few treatments available were pretty low tech, the cost of treatment was not much of a factor for middle class couples. Baby-producing options beyond treatment were clear, too. There were two. Donor insemination was available for some couples. Most couples, however, were steered towards adoption of a baby. Adoptable babies were readily available in a time when sex outside of marriage was a reality but reliable birth control was not, where abortion was illegal and dangerous and single parenthood was considered shameful.

A generation later, for Dave and me, there were several more treatment options, but fewer adoption options. In our first round of treatment, though, there was nothing specific that could be done about our identified problem: hopelessly blocked fallopian tubes. Surgery was tried but failed. Our infertility appeared hopelessly permanent. We were devastated. As children raised in the '50s and told we could have anything if we worked hard enough, we were also angry. Only one good thing was apparent: at least our medical insurance covered almost everything we had undergone. We eventually realized that what we wanted most was to be parents, and so, after waiting a couple of years, we adopted in the middle 1970s. By the early '80s when we had become increasingly anxious about expanding our family, everything had changed! In vitro fertilization was available, but not particularly successful. Adoption was less available and increasingly complicated. Ultimately, after many complications, we added two more children to our family.

Now, our oldest child is a young adult. If, in the next few years, he and a partner decide to grow a family and find themselves to be infertile, they will face an alphabet soup of expensive and invasive testing and treatment options and powerful drugs. Current treatments that have created much greater statistical likelihood of pregnancy for the late Boomers and Generation X carry with them a dangerous (to both mother and baby) and stressful potential side effect: a significant risk of a multiple pregnancy. What's more, because successful treatment often involves using discoveries from rapidly advancing research, insurers try to define more and more treatments as "experimental" so that they can refuse to cover them financially. Complicating the mix are the moral and ethical dilemmas introduced by collaborative reproductive options which involve the genetic material or reproductive capacities of people outside the marriage and the possibility of using selective abortion to "reduce" a multiple gestation to safter numbers. At the same time adoption is much more complicated and more expensive and involves many more options than ever before.

No, it's never been like this before.

THE EMOTIONAL SIDE EFFECTS

In 1973 a Boston area nurse-midwife who had personally faced infertility, Barbara Eck Menning, founded a local support group for those experiencing infertility. She named it RESOLVE, a name chosen to reflect the purpose of the group: to help couples reach the resolution stage of grieving the pain of being infertile. This was all quite revolutionary. Before Barbara Menning infertility had always been a closeted issue. Nobody talked about it and nobody wrote about it. Because it was linked to sex, it somehow was considered shameful.

8

Barbara Eck Menning opened a closet door and let in the light of new thinking. For the first time it was suggested that the medical conditions that produced infertility had emotional side effects that nobody was talking about, and that by acknowledging that infertility produced a grief reaction—first surprise, then denial and bargaining, often isolation and despair, and finally resolution—couples dealing with this process could be helped to feel whole again.

Barbara's was an idea whose time had come, and today RESOLVE—which has grown far beyond just being a support group to being an education, referral and advocacy source for the infertile—has substantially over 50 chapters throughout the United States. RESOLVE's success has encouraged the formation of similar groups in other countries. IAAC, the Infertility Awareness Association of Canada, for example, operates with a chapter system very similarly to RESOLVE. INCIID, The InterNational Council on Infertility Information Dissemination is an internet-based source for education, information and support. In some communities doctors or hospitals or houses of worship sponsor local support groups.

It is generally accepted by the professional community today that while infertility only rarely has emotional causes, it almost always has emotional side effects. Let's talk about some...

TURNING POINTS AND LOSSES

With or without infertility, as we move though our lives we go through a series of turning points. Some have called these crossroads, passages, or life crises. No matter what terminology is used, the situation described is the same: these are the periods in each person's individual development or in the growth of a couple which find them exceptionally vulnerable to the gains and losses which are a part of the ebb and flow of life. Each of these turning points finds us giving up some familiarly comfortable assumptions about ourselves in order to allow for inner growth. Beyond each of these turning points we find our lives permanently restructured in both positive and negative ways.

The passage of infertility demands that a couple give up an assumption that has been with them since childhood, when they began to hear and to assimilate such casual comments as, "Well, Jenny (or Jimmy), when you are a mommy (or daddy) you can do it your way." With us from our childhoods has been the assumption that we would, if we wanted to, someday be the parents of a child conceived in the love we feel for another human being we've chosen to be our life's partner.

Another way to look at such an experience might be as a "non event." In their book *Going to Plan B: How You Can Cope, Regroup, and Start Your Life on a New Path*, Nancy K. Schlossberg and Susan Porter Robinson define a non event as an event which didn't happen in one's life

9

but which one reasonably could expect would happen, so that it's absence changed one's life. The appearance of a non-event in our lives demands that we make adjustments, balance disappointments, reframe our goals. Examples of non-events that change people's lives might include not being admitted to the school you had expected to attend, or working very hard for a promotion ultimately given to someone else, or not being offered a professional basketball contract though you'd played very well in college... or not being able to give birth to the number of children you'd planned to have.

For most couples parenthood no longer happens by chance, but instead, after deliberate decision making to determine whether parenting is for them, couples consciously stop using birth control, buy ovulation predictors, and make serious efforts to conceive. When, after several months of fruitless efforts, a couple is faced with the possibility of giving up control over their life planning, as well as the personal magic of their long-held expectations that they could and would become parents, most couples who find themselves dealing with impaired fertility at first find it difficult to admit to themselves that there is indeed a problem and to allow themselves to experience the full impact of their emotions. So for some couples, infertility begins with a long period of denial. ("We're busy people and we're missing the 'right' day"... "My partner travels so often on business." etc.)

Many people assume that getting a baby—by birth or by adoption—is the resolution to infertility. But this is not what resolution is. Feelings about infertility don't necessarily go away with the arrival of a much-wanted child in the home of a couple who has been working toward this goal for a long time. In fact, for some people feelings accompanying infertility don't necessarily ever go away.

Pregnancy is a physical goal which is achievable by 70% of infertile couples. Parenting is a life role objective possible for still more couples who choose alternative routes to parenthood. But resolution is an emotional goal. It is the ongoing process of first coming to grips with the reality that the physical goal of a jointly conceived child may be difficult or even impossible to achieve and then confronting this reality head on and dealing with the resulting stress this will bring to each individual and to the couple as a unit. Resolution is a process of growth and change involving making decisions about options and alternatives in ways that are positive and productive. It is accomplished in degrees over time, so that identifying one couple as resolved and another as not is seldom possible or realistic. The goal toward which resolving infertile couples are working is the ability to incorporate both the gains and the losses that infertility will bring to their lives into a positive image of themselves as individuals and of the two of them as a family.

No, it isn't just a baby infertile people risk losing. The infertility experience is even more complicated than that. Infertility involves the potential for multiple losses, including, but not limited to the following...

Perhaps most clearly and immediately felt by those of us who experience infertility is the **loss of control** over numerous aspects of our lives. Today's couple, who came to sexual maturity and selected a partner after the birth control revolution precipitated by the wide availability of the birth control pill in the mid sixties, have always had the distinct expectation that they would be able to control their fertility. Unfortunately, because infertility was not discussed as they grew up, this expectation included not just the belief that they would be able to avoid pregnancy when they so desired, but that they would be able to achieve pregnancy when they so desired.

Naive as it may seem in retrospect, most people begin the journey toward parenthood with plans like these: "We'll get pregnant in September so that the baby will be born in May and I'll have time to get back into my bikini by summer," or "You can go off birth control right in the spring before we get our degrees and then take the board exams in the summer before your pregnancy starts to show." Losing control of a part of life which their peers take so completely for granted is devastating and, for many people, precipitates a humiliating blow to self esteem.

And this loss of control takes on an even greater dimension now, at the turn of a new century, than it did a decade or two ago. According to Judith D. Schwartz, in a June 29, 1993 *New York Times* article "The New Mommy Trap,"

"Reproduction has taken on a new cachet, and savvy marketers have taken note. In advertising, fantasy has traditionally implied sexual imagery, unattainable luxury or exotic settings. The new message is that the nuclear family is better than all that...Reproduction (implicitly meaning biological parenthood) has become a trope for individual success."

Schwartz goes on to point out that recently advertisers have begun to take this tack in promoting everything from ovulation detectors to fragrances (DNA, Eternity, etc.) to clothing (The Gap) and food products (Tyson Chicken.) The resulting implication that controlled family building is the ultimate sign of success creates extraordinary pressure on the one in six couples experiencing a fertility impairment.

Yet treating infertility demands that couples give up even more control. Control of their sexual privacy and spontaneity, for example, is forfeited to a medical team which asks them to chart their intercourse, supply semen samples, appear within hours after intercourse for a post-coital test, etc. Months of counting days, reading basal thermometers before our eyes are even in focus in the morning, plotting little x's on a graph to represent when we had intercourse (and sometimes wondering with some embarrassment whether we should add a couple so that the doctor won't think we're not "really trying"!) takes its toll. Couples who explore adoption often complain that they feel that they've lost control of other areas usually seen as private (discussion of their sex lives, access to their income tax forms, etc.) to a social worker or attorney or to prospective birthparents.

Control of calendars is given over to treatment. An ill-timed out-of-town business trip can ruin a whole month's chances for conception. A social invitation to share a rustic and noisy cabin for the weekend involves a check to see whether the date falls on a "fertile weekend."

Many infertility treatments involve therapy with various hormones which may, along with the general stress of being a "patient," contribute to massive mood swings and shifts, making both patient and partner feel out of control of emotions. Too often, patients have too little information and develop unrealistic expectations about their ability to control these shifts. They become angry and ashamed of their inability to exert control over their emotional reactions and they may isolate themselves from others.

What type or size car to buy depends on whether or not it will be carrying children. Accepting a new job or a promotion can become dependent on how travel impacts on the treatment program, whether or not the new company has excellent health care benefits which cover infertility treatments, as well as whether or not the new employee's coverage for infertility treatment would be excluded because it was defined by the insurance company as a pre-existing condition. Continuing education may be put on hold when a woman expects that any day she will become pregnant, so that finishing a term might be difficult or impossible. Whether to buy a house in the suburbs with sidewalks for Big Wheels or a condo in the city close to work and cultural events is controlled by infertility. Even the most private and seemingly simple of decisions—how much time to spend in a hot tub, how much coffee to drink, how many miles to run each week, whether to buy briefs or boxer shorts—can be controlled by the infertility experience.

Couples often comment that with infertility they feel that they have lost control of <u>every</u> aspect of their lives. To many individuals for whom being in control is an important part of their ability to feel confident and competent, infertility represents a devastating loss... but this is not infertility's only loss.

Potentially, infertility means the **loss of our individual genetic continuity**—our expectation that we will continue the genes of our families in an unbroken blood line from some distant past into a promising future. For those raised in blood-is-thicker-than-water cultures, this loss is significant enough to be avoided at nearly any cost.

Genetic connection seems to be less important in general among people who are several generations removed from their immigrant grandparents in "melting pot" or "patchwork quilt" cultures such as that of the U.S., Canada, and Australia. And as we become a more transient world, wherein large numbers of people live far removed from their families of origin, it has become increasingly accepted that people build kinship communities which substitute for genetic families from among the people with whom they feel a common bond. Still, in many countries, in many ethnic communities, in some religions, and in many families, genetic connection remains a cultural imperative! Why we feel this way is not so important as is the fact that we acknowledge that we do indeed feel this way. And for infertile individuals for whom this loss is central and powerful, pursuing family building alternatives which allow only one partner to retain genetic continuity can be devastating to some relationships.

Some families are entirely comfortable with the idea of adopting in order to carry a family into the future, while others believe strongly that the family blood line cannot be grafted onto. Moreover, as a whole, society defines parent-child relationships primarily by blood ties, and clearly devalues as second-best or second-rate any parent-child relationships which do not include genetic connection such as those in adoption, stepparenting, fostering, mentoring. We are fascinated in a macabre way by stories of babies switched at birth, fathers who discover that the children they were parenting were in fact products of adultery, adoptees who murder their parents. Adopters are frequently asked if they have any children "of their own" or comforted that it is "too bad that they don't." It can be frightening to consider that in order to have the parenting experience we may need to accept a "social handicap" in this role and deal with being seen as "odd" for a lifetime.

And the loss of our genetic continuity is not just our own loss. For some, to experience this loss means to let one's family down. More than just offering our parents the social opportunity to be grandparents, some infertile people fear that being unable to carry forward the family's genes may cause them to be seen as failures or disappointments to their parents or grandparents.

Our dreams about parenting included the expectation of our parenting a jointly conceived child. In choosing a life's partner all of us do at least a little fantasizing about what our children might be like. Will he have her intellect and his sense of humor? Grandpa's red hair and Aunt Wilma's athletic prowess? Gosh, think of the medical expenses if she inherits both her mother's crossed eye and her father's terrible overbite!

For some, accepting the **loss of a jointly conceived child** means little more than throwing away the romantic notions fed by years of movies and novels in favor of what we define as a more practical and realistic view of relationships. But for others, this dreamed-of child who represents the blending of both the best and the worst of our most intimate selves also represents a kind of ultimate intimacy—an eternal bonding of partner to partner. After all, in giving our genes to one another for blending, we offer our most vulnerable and intimate and valuable sense of ourselves—a gift that is perhaps the most precious we can offer. Losing that dream and so feeling forced to consider alternatives such as donor insemination, hiring a surrogate mother, adopting, etc. can be painful indeed for those for whom this expectation was particularly important.

There is also the loss of the **physical satisfactions of the pregnancy and birth experiences.** Many people see the loss of a pregnancy as belonging entirely to women, but this is not true. Though the physical changes and challenges of pregnancy and birth are experienced by women alone, producing a child, as any counselor of pregnant teens will verify, is the ultimate rite of passage for both men and women—the final mark of having reached adulthood. You're grown up now, man, and your parents aren't in charge anymore. Beyond that, the physical ability to impregnate a woman or to carry and birth a child represents the ultimate expression of maleness or femaleness—our bodies at work doing what they were built to do. For many people, losing such capacities challenges their feelings about their maturity or their sexuality or both—about their competence as adult men and women. And to make it worse for couples of the '80s and '90s, an era when physical fitness has achieved almost a cult-like status, the loss of physical expectations about becoming or making pregnant may represent an even more deeply felt loss of body image than it did for couples just a half generation older.

Such feelings are rooted in societal expectations. It is their own discomfort with and fear of the loss of the physical aspects of getting/making pregnant which generates from outsiders the tasteless humor which relates infertility to sexuality in comments such as, "Do you need a little help there? Happy to offer my services!" or "Let me show you how it's done." or "Hey, all Steve has to do is look at me and I'm pregnant. It must be something in the water!"

And then there are the **emotional gratifications of a shared pregnancy, prepared childbirth, breast-feeding experience** which were a part of our expectations about having children. Over the last two decades, a substantial element of our society, fearful of the impact of massive changes in family structure, has mysticized the experience of birth to an exaggerated extent. In search of the perfect "bonding" experience (billed as a kind of magical super glue without which many fear that families will disintegrate) couples carefully choose specific kinds of childbirth preparation, attend classes together, read books, practice breathing, etc. They expect to experience a magical closeness in spousal relationships, an irreplaceable wonder in sharing the birth experience, an instant eye-to-eye bonding between parents and child. Hospitals market to the expectations of these couples in expensively done and romantically scripted television commercials and display ads. They compete with one another to provide perfect preparation and birthing rooms with the perfect equipment (birthing beds, chairs, tanks) and the perfect atmosphere (music, guests allowed, champagne after, etc.) Certainly the newest pronatalist advertising trend Judith Schwartz has identified, which urges parenthood on both sexes, welcoming men to the "fun" and tuning in to women's reproductive anxieties about timing, is simply a new twist on the same old theme.

This set of expectations about the emotional gratifications of a shared pregnancy, prepared childbirth, breast-feeding experience, though far too often unrealistic, is widely held, and may contribute to our own unrecognized prejudices about family life. To risk losing such an experience is much more significant to today's couple than it would have been to their parents and grandparents—many of whose mothers gave birth anesthetized in sterile operating rooms while fathers paced in waiting rooms outside, who often didn't see and hold their children until hours after their births, who bottle-fed formula to their infants (but who did indeed manage to bond with us, their children!)

And finally, to be permanently infertile threatens one with the **loss of the opportunity to parent,** which is a major developmental goal for most adults. The psychologist Eric Erickson has identified a series of developmental milestones humans work toward throughout the life span. In adulthood, the major goals are regenerativity and parenting. To be infertile, on the surface, threatens our ability to achieve that goal, so that for many people this represents a devastating blow.

Erickson and others have clearly demonstrated that it is possible for individuals to achieve the developmental goal and to satisfy the need for parenting without actually becoming biological or legal parents. Many adults find ways of redirecting or rechanneling their need to nurture—through interaction with nieces and nephews and family friends; by choosing work which brings them in frequent contact with children; by volunteering as religious class teachers, scout leaders, or for a group such as Big Brothers/Big Sisters; by becoming active in non-child centered volunteer work; by nurturing the earth through nature hobbies such as gardening, etc.

This is not to imply that lists of possible redirections like these are seen as equivalent substitutions or as realistic direct replacements for the lifelong experience of parenting a child jointly conceived and birthed with a much loved partner. Please don't suggest anything like that to your infertile friend! While some adults can and do actively choose to meet their developmental needs to nurture without becoming parents, for couples who have once made the choice to become parents and have then been thwarted by infertility, the choice to redirect that energy is much more difficult. But the exploration of such options is an important part of addressing this loss. Marianne Takas and Edward Warner wrote the valuable book *To Love a Child* (Addison Wesley, 1992) as a way to seriously examine for themselves options for satisfying these nurturing needs.

It is all of these six potential and realized losses and others related to them which tear at the gut during those days or weeks or months when couples tried to deny the infertility. These losses are the danger lurking in the crisis, and they are difficult to face. Facing feelings about infertility's losses can help couples find the opportunities in the crisis and in deciding what treatment, what lifestyle alternative is right for them. And facing the emotional ramifications of infertility will help infertile couples to make

15

better decisions about its practical aspects. But facing those emotional ramifications can also be frightening. Infertile couples need understanding friends and family during this time.

SURPRISE AND DENIAL: A PATTERN BEGINS

Keeping in mind that all of the things that make us unique individuals—our genetic and cultural heritages, the family and the town and the schools and the religion in which we grew up, our talents and weaknesses, our life experiences, etc.—also make us experience infertility uniquely, there is still a pattern of reacting to such a life crisis. Learning to recognize the steps in that pattern can help those experiencing the crisis and those who are trying to help them to deal with it.

<u>Surprised</u> (because, after all, how could birth control generation people be infertile?) many couples tend to deny that there could be a problem for a while. Soon couples may find their surprise tinged with embarrassment as the questions begin...

"Hey, when are you two gonna start a family? Mom and I have been waiting for some grandkids. Uncle Harry and Aunt Alice have four!"...or

"Hey, Jamal, no kids yet? Are ya doin' it right? Need a little advice or maybe a demonstration? Ha, ha, ha."

Perhaps they're just trying too hard. Perhaps they're hitting the wrong day (after all, they have such busy lives and Terry <u>is</u> out of town a lot.) <u>Denial</u> is a kind of safety mechanism that the mind creates when dealing with a potentially explosive problem. And a short stretch of denial is not necessarily unhealthy. Denial allows one time to muster coping resources. But continuing to deny reality pushes both physical and emotional resolution farther into the future, and, unfortunately, denial can be unproductively reinforced by people like you, who, in trying to be comforting, offer inaccurate advice such as, "Honey, just relax. You and Bob are trying too hard. You need to take a vacation. I guarantee you'll come home pregnant."

It's hard to relax when you think that not relaxing is going to keep you from getting pregnant. And besides, normal tension is not a cause of infertility; it is the result of it.

Unfortunately, denial is sometimes reinforced by the first professional the couple seeks out. Too often a family doctor will respond to an awkward query about trying to get pregnant by reminding a couple that they are still young and suggesting they give it more time. The fact is that it takes an average couple less than six months to conceive, and 85% of couples trying to achieve a pregnancy do so within a year. For the other

16

15%, the likelihood is that they are not going to conceive without some sort of medical intervention.

More trying, more tension, no results, bad advice. Wrote Dan Clements in a RESOLVE of Maryland newsletter years ago, "It never ceases to amaze me how much other people deny our infertility ...relax, take a cruise... don't worry about it... pray...donate money to charity...stop thinking about it so much..." It is interesting to note that when my friend Howie got cancer no one advised the above as possible cures for his condition. All of the advice is friendly... but none of it is relevant to infertility. It all contains a basic assumption that is a lie—that infertility is caused by something other than medical causes."

Sometimes this well meaning advice seems on the surface too practical to discard.

"Hey, you oughta see my guy, Dr. Blank. He's a specialist. On the wall of his examining room is a plaque from the American Society for Reproductive Medicine. Why, it says right on the door 'Obstetrics, Gynecology, Infertility.'"

It is usually a very good idea to start working on infertility with one's own gynecologist. Infertility is indeed part of the general training every obstetrician/gynecologist and urologist takes to become certified in his or her own specialty. If the couple is fortunate, the doctor with whom they begin will be among a number of ob/gyns who practice infertility in a sensitive manner. Such doctors are careful to schedule infertility patients so that they can avoid contact with obstetrics patients. The practice usually includes an associate or a specially trained nurse clinician who can see the infertility patient in need of a timely test or treatment when the primary physician is called away from the office to deliver a baby.

However, not all gynecologists do practice infertility in such a sensitive manner. While experts in infertility generally concur that a basic workup which will reveal all possible problems a couple has (and often there is more than one problem) can and should be completed in three to six months, a great many doctors insist on one test at a time, menstrual cycle after unproductive menstrual cycle, offer unwarranted treatments, and allow months and months of unproductive visits without either completing all tests or suggesting referral to more expert help. Even now, at the turn of a new century, many doctors who are not infertility specialists will not suggest the simplest, least invasive and least expensive test of all—a man's sperm analysis—until several months and many tests after first seeing a woman.

Sooner rather than later couples who begin with a general practice physician or a general ob/gyn probably should change doctors. The subspecialty areas of gynecology (called reproductive endocrinology and infertility) and of urology (called andrology) are rapidly growing fields. In 1980 there were fewer than 75 of such specialists in the entire United

States, but today there are hundreds. Only the most remotely rural areas are not within a four hour drive of genuinely specialized care.

But as much as you care about this couple, you are not likely to be in a position to know the correct timing for such a switch or to suggest the most appropriate practitioner. Instead, what you can and should do is to make certain that the couple is aware of the existence of the infertility group closest to them for referral. If there is no local group nearby, put them in touch with the national office of RESOLVE (in the United States) or of IAAC (Infertility Awareness Association of Canada) or with INCIID. If the couple is already in close contact with such an organization, back off, please. You may safely assume that they are very well aware of their own doctor's qualifications as they compare with others within a reasonable distance, and you should not question their good judgment in this area.

It is their frustration with well meant but inaccurate advice that often initiates another stage in the grieving pattern— isolation.

TOGETHER ALONE

Confronted by blooming trees and bulging bellies of a fertile world, the infertile couple sometimes needs to isolate themselves. Everyone around them is getting pregnant. Some friends are having reproductive accidents about which they complain loud and long. Too many activities seem impossibly centered on family and constantly remind them of the children which elude them.

Much of what they are experiencing now you truly cannot understand. Tears, jealousy about one's sister's new baby, hatred of pregnant strangers in the grocery store are all normal reactions to infertility, though experiencing such reactions makes infertile people feel terribly guilty. They need you to understand that unpredictable and inconsistent avoidance of office baby showers or family christenings, their possible unwillingness to share in family holiday celebrations, are not examples of what you may have perceived as selfishness or irrational moodiness. The isolation of infertile people is instead a necessary self-protective part of the resolution process. If you cannot understand and support at least with quiet tolerance the need of an infertile couple to pull back, you will have rejected them at a time during which they most need to know that someone understands; and should you choose to confront them angrily with your judgment that they are being "childish" or "selfish" you will risk permanent damage to your relationship.

Alone, the infertile couple will deal with particularly difficult issues. Each of them is likely to be in pain and dealing with individual losses. No matter which partner received the medical diagnosis of a fertility impairment, both partners, since they love one another and see each other as permanent partners, face the possible loss of their reproductive powers. It may seen natural for you to try to offer help to the "sick" one, but you must be careful to remember that by virtue of the diagnosis <u>both</u> of these people are infertile and need your support.

A couple's sexuality, already battered by an unspontaneous and totally unromantic routine of ovulation prediction, invasive and uncomfortable tests, and scheduled intercourse, may be called into question. With spontaneity gone, many couples experience a time when all interest in sex is lost for a time. An unplanned and undiscussed moratorium may be called. Since it is unlikely that both partners will have reached this point at the same time, a sudden loss of interest in sex by one partner may frighten the other. If this point comes during treatment, it may produce resentment, as one spouse may feel that the other is undermining treatment. If it occurs after treatment has stopped, it may generate the panicky fear that being infertile means being asexual.

Are they going to mention any of this to you? Probably not! Does infertility cause marital stress? You bet!

LASHING OUT

Anger is a particularly common by-product of both the stress of infertility testing and treatment and the losses which accompany it. At whom that anger is directed is unpredictable. The target could be a doctor or nurse, a marriage partner, a co-worker, God, a social worker, fertile friends, Mom or Dad—maybe you!

Some of this anger may be justified and rational, the result of insensitivity or of invaded privacy or of hearing just one too many pieces of misguided advice. But sometimes an explosive venting of frustration and disappointment and exhaustion just catches a caring other being at the wrong place at the wrong time.

All of us have limited resources. We have just so much money, just so much time, just so much physical energy, so much emotional reserves. Infertility drains away huge chunks of all of these resources, leaving infertile people feeling frayed and abandoned. Of course I'm going to ask you to be patient with your infertile friend. But I'm also going to tell you that you shouldn't allow yourself to be scapegoated. Furthermore, people in crisis do sometimes become blinded and can benefit from a dose of compassionate reality.

If you feel a need to confront the infertile person in your life, choose a private time rather than a public forum to address this issue with your friend. Be honest, but try to remain as calm as you can in explaining your own pain or confusion about the anger. Try not to be defensive if your friend points out that you have been insensitive. Admit your inexperience and ask for information or clarification. Then allow your friend space and come back again soon to offer support.

What infertile couples would like most from you or from me or from someone, anyway ("the experts," perhaps?) is a magic formula which would make their problem go away, taking with it the discomfort and eventually the anguish and substituting the long sought pregnancy. But there is no magic formula.

As a friend, what you can do for a couple stuck in this spot is to offer them informed understanding and support from the base of your already built caring relationship with them. An infertility support group can offer help for both you and them. Such groups will offer you accurate information to reinforce your interest in being compassionately helpful. The groups can help the infertile to identify the sources of their medical problems and emotional discomfort and the tools for dealing with these from the base of the empathetic understanding of one who has also been there.

This isolation and anger you've noticed in your infertile friends comes because they are immersed in that predictable course of grieving we've been working through: shock/surprise, denial, isolation, rage/anger, bargaining, sadness/depression, and finally resolution. These are the stages in grieving any loss, whether it be a child's mourning for the loss of his favorite toy left on the plane to Grandma's or the adolescent's loss of her first love or the young adult's not being hired for the dream job or a grandparent's dying.

Infertility's grief reaction may, on close inspection, look more like the big time grieving that accompanies death or other major loss, but sometimes it's hard to recognize that. With infertility there has been no "sickness," there is no body to prepare, to funeral to arrange, so that the chances are good that friends and family may not recognize their loved ones as mourners.

In fact, sometimes the couple themselves will take a long to recognize that they are grieving. One of the reasons this is true is that each of the partners—and sometimes their family members, too—may be experiencing grief about a different one of infertility's losses discussed earlier. While one partner's anger and sadness may be over the loss of the pregnancy experience, for example, the other may be railing against feeling so out of control. At the same time, would-be grandparents may be mourning their family's loss of genetic continuity. They're sharing a situation in common, and yet their personal grief reactions are different enough that they may feel unable to offer appropriate comfort to one another or they may be unable to find helpful the consolation which is offered.

SADNESS, DEPRESSION AND MOVING ON...

Depression and deep sadness are an inescapable part of a grief cycle, and the cyclical nature of infertility treatment—two weeks of hope followed by crashing despair when the period comes—contributes to a building sadness that eventually seems to permeate every aspect of an infertile couple's lives together.

Even couples who fall into the 50-70% of couples who ultimately do become pregnant and deliver a child genetically related to both of them are likely to have experienced this sadness and depression, but for those who must eventually face the probability that they will not conceive together, this particular sadness and depression is very much like mourning a death—in this case the death of dreams and expectations. Those who try to adopt and come close but lose an opportunity have much in common emotionally with those who experience a miscarriage—a situation rarely acknowledged by caring others.

Depression brings with it some lethargy and despair—a pervasive feeling of distress. There may be irrational behavior changes, a loss of appetite and subsequent weight loss, inability to sleep. There will likely be a great deal of emotional drifting, and all of the grief stricken person's earlier experienced emotions will seem to crash back in, as the griever feels angry, guilty, out of control.

Now is the time when an infertile couple will truly mourn for the child they had logically assumed would come one day—the child whose face they had each begun to conjure somewhere in their childhoods. This child who would have had all of the good and bad genetic traits of his parents and grandparents— Grandpa's crooked grin, Dad's eyes, Mom's sense of humor—will need to be buried. Buried with him will be an assortment of related dreams—a wife's fantasy of how she might tell her husband of their miracle pregnancy, their shared fantasy of how they would tell others, the dream of going through prepared childbirth classes and a perfect Lamaze delivery—all of these dreams will need to be released.

During this most wrenching emotional experience of letting go, an infertile couple will need the support of their family and friends more than ever. It will be difficult for them to see, however, when they are so blinded by their own grief, how deeply the finality of their infertility may affect their families. For families, too, may grieve for lost assumptions—for the grandchildren, nieces and nephews not to be born. The continuation of an unbroken genetic lines is very important to many people. Parents of an infertile couple, in particular, often   find themselves writhing in guilt—finding ways to attempt to blame themselves for their children's physical problems. If these grieving people could only identify one another as mourners, their shared grief could be worked through together with mutual support to ease each one's very personal pain. But this is often a difficult to impossible recognition.

21

It is never easy to work through a grieving process. Grievers may feel that life can't go on, that nothing will ever be the same again. Since the grief of infertility is often silent and unacknowledged, since too often the tears and moodiness are judged with impatience rather than understood and expected, the burial of dreams can move slowly. This process does, however, almost always give way with time to the slow but steady return of a basic optimism for the future and a realization that, as in any life crisis with its attendant gains and losses, life has been permanently altered, but that it can and will go on... and eventually happily.

This regained ability to feel optimism and to accept the losses of infertility as both a positive and a negative in our lives is the beginning of resolution. RESOLVE's founder, Barbara Eck Menning, framed it best in her book *Infertility: A Guide for the Childless Couple*:

My infertility resides in my heart like an old friend. I do not hear from it for weeks at a time, and then, a moment, a thought, a baby announcement or some such thing... and I will feel the tug—maybe even be sad or shed a few tears. And I think, "There's my old friend." It will always be a part of me.

GETTING STUCK

Resolution is the goal. With it comes the ability to clearly and carefully re-examine options—alternative routes to parenthood like adoption or collaborative reproduction, alternative lifestyles like childfree living. But it's not uncommon for infertile people to get a little stuck in one of grief's stages before they are able to move on. Some couples deny the fertility impairment for a really long time before getting into effective treatment. Others deny that they could ever be negative statistics, and so, in this era when there has never been more fast moving research, they get caught up in the conveyor belt of treatment and seem completely incapable of stopping. Others get stuck in anger—and because it's safer to rage against someone other than a marriage partner, family members or friends may be convenient (sometimes irrational, sometimes appropriate) targets of that anger. Still others spend a long time in the "if-only" stage of grief called bargaining. ("If only we had started trying sooner."... "If only we'd not tried to save our money first.")

In their grief, the infertile couple may dredge up the past, working through guilty thoughts in an attempt to find a spiritual reason for their infertility. Those raised in the Judeo-Christian tradition may know the stories of Hannah, Rachel, Sarah, Leah, and Elizabeth, all of whom, after years of infertility, finally became pregnant. Through theologians make clear that finding of favor with God is not the key to success in any of these stories, many times they are misinterpreted in this way. ("If I promise to be good from now on, God, will you make me pregnant?") Logic is often absent in a time of crisis, so attempts to explain this may prove fruitless. It may take a great deal of time for the infertile couple—perhaps even for you—to recognize that fertility is not a reward for being good while infertility is a punishment for being bad.

When you're stuck, it's hard to move on, and it's hard to consider other options, and it's easy to begin to feel obsessed with the infertility to the extent that it appears to overwhelm daily life and thinking and all conversations.

What is most difficult about obsession is that it may block healthy resolution by short circuiting logic. It is when they are obsessed with infertility that a couple may begin to think that resolution means getting a child, from any source, as quickly as possible, and at whatever physical, emotional, or financial cost necessary. Being obsessed may mean asking to remain on high levels of powerful drugs which have been unproductive for them after their physicians feel that they have passed the point of good medical practice. Obsession may mean volunteering for a fourth or fifth or seventh GIFT of ICSI cycle, though the odds for success seem abysmally low. A couple who is obsessed will not recognize that it may be time to stop treatment. On the other hand, they are not ready to deal with most of infertility's alternatives, either.

These couples race an inner clock and are desperately eager to get on with life after infertility's often lengthy stall. Stopping or taking a break is particularly hard for 40-something couples to do. Facing taking time out to consider carefully the pros and cons of any new treatment or any family-building alternative seems impossible. The issue of control rears its head again. Angry that their goals have been thwarted, an obsessive couple may wish to by-pass the lengthy institutionalized adoption system primarily because they resent the homestudy process and view it not as a healthy opportunity for objective growth and preparation, but as another example of someone other than themselves being in control of their lives. After seeing a news report about a calamity in another country they may suddenly, and without apparent preparation or previous thought, race to adopt children who become suddenly "available." Such a couple is primed to be victimized by a potentially illegal black market adoption, because they cannot discern the difference between this and an ethically handled private placement. Obsessive couples refuse to look at donor insemination or embryo transfer as <u>alternatives</u> to their infertility but prefer to think of them as "medicines" that cure it. They may be unprepared, then, to deal with the losses which accompany building families with donor gametes and their life-long impact on their own lives and the lives of children so conceived. Obsessive couples refuse to listen to or to respond to long term concerns or societal objections to various treatment options. They reject the idea of a need for "preparation" for any of these alternative routes to parenthood.

Obsessive couples more than couples who have worked through and resolved their infertility-related grief may find a subsequent pregnancy

23

and birth experience less satisfying than their expectations had led them to believe that they would be. Often such couples have unrealistic expectations of their children by birth or adoption. Often they deny for extended periods the realities of the alternatives they have leapt into without completing the resolution process.

It isn't just the infertile couples' own unmet needs that feed an obsession, nor is it only the confusion about when to stop treatment that is generated by proliferating research. Pressure comes, too, from family and friends. Often without meaning to, loved ones send messages that indicate their own disappointment in a couple's infertility problems and their own lack of acceptance of the alternatives available to the infertile couple. Even silence can be misinterpreted by the infertile couple as indicative of disappointment. Such messages heighten the couple's guilty feelings and increase their fear that reproductive failure will let the family down. Careful, direct communication, rather than avoidance of the painful issues, is imperative if such mixed messages are to be avoided.

If you suspect that the infertile couple you care about is stuck obsessively in one of infertility's stages, try gently to guide them toward counseling. However, not just any counselor works well with infertile people. An infertility self help group will help them find appropriate counseling through their own support groups, or beyond them to clergy, family therapists, psychologists, clinic social workers, etc. whom the group has identified as sensitive to the uniqueness of the infertility experience.

PREGNANT... BUT STILL INFERTILE??

Most fertility impaired couples who begin the grieving process we have described will go through all of its stages. However, since a majority of couples—over 50%—are truly impaired fertiles rather than permanently infertile, most will eventually become pregnant.

At the announcement of a pregnancy, the logical reaction from you, the friends of this couple, would be relief, elation, and an expectation that now all would be well with the world for this couple. You would likely expect that their tension would lift, the introspection would dissipate, and there would be a happily-ever-after ending to their story.

For couples whose experience with fertility impairment has been relatively brief, a pregnancy may indeed be enthusiastically welcomed and enjoyed to the fullest. A pregnancy for a couple who have spent a long time in fertility studies and treatment, however, usually is not the experience about which they fantasized. Many couples find it difficult to relate to the "normally fertile" world. Some experience high risk pregnancies, and, even for those whose pregnancies are not at high risk, there may be heightened anxiety levels throughout the pregnancy and even for a time after the baby's birth. After all, such couples reason, their bodies were faulty and betrayed them before. How could they expect anything other than the worst?

24

There are several stages of a pregnancy that may be particularly difficult for such a couple. The first is validating the pregnancy and accepting it as a reality. Another is coming to accept the baby as a part of the mother's body and preparing for the physical changes a pregnancy will bring. A third difficult stage may be fetal distinction—coming to see the baby not just as a growth changing the shape of its mother, but as a separate distinct person who will actually be born and thus needs to be planned for. Lastly, those who have experienced infertility may find it difficult to allow themselves to prepare actively for a role transition from non-parent to parent.

Your flexible support and your realistic, rather than romantic, attitude about the pregnancy and birth experience and subsequent parenting are important to the pregnant infertile couple. You should understand that for a long time this pregnancy may not make them feel any less infertile than before. Having already separated themselves from what they perceive as the "normal" world, but embarrassed to appear ungrateful to you and their still infertile friends, these couples may feel lost in a kind of limbo. They need all of your careful understanding and support.

OTHER DOORS...

Helen Keller wrote
"When one door of happiness closes, another opens, But often we look so long at the closed door that we do not see the one that has opened for us. We must all find these open doors, and if we believe in ourselves we will find them, and make ourselves and our lives as beautiful as God intended."

This poignant description of resolution to loss has been helpful to many infertile people looking beyond infertility to other doors to happiness.

Whether because the medical problem appears to be irreversible or because they've simply reached a point where they are ready to expend their financial and physical and emotional energies differently, many infertile couples decide to explore other models of family life. The healthiest way for infertile couples to look at alternatives from collaborative reproduction to adoption to childfree living is to step back and reexamine the original decision to have children and to determine whether infertility has had a changing effect on that original decision.

The infertile couple may choose to remain childless but to do so not with unhappy resignation (perhaps the easy way out, as it involves no more difficult decision making) but instead with optimistic decisiveness—regaining control and making a choice to become childfree. Since they will have at one time made a decision to have children (and probably announced that decision to their private world of friends and family) going back to reexamine the childfree option may seem incongruous and even outrageous to an infertile couple at first. However, living childfree has numerous advantages. For some couples the advantages of this alternative will far outweigh the advantages of the alternative ways to become parents. A couple re-exploring this alternative will find Mike and Jean Carter's *Sweet Grapes: How to Stop Being Infertile and Start Living Again* (Perspectives Press, 1989) helpful, and so might you.

A second alternative the infertile couple may wish to explore is choosing to parent a child who is biologically one spouse's and is, in essence, adopted by the other. These are the options referred to earlier as collaborative reproduction, because they result from a collaboration between an infertile couple and one or more fertile people willing to help them in their quest to have a baby. In addition to the general infertility support groups, advocacy groups which serve these families—and will be happy to provide accurate information to you, as well—include OPTS (The Organization of Parents through Surrogacy) and The Alliance for Donor Insemination Families.

Donor insemination, which involves using a catheter or syringe to place the sperm of a fertile male into the reproductive tract of the wife is the procedure such a couple would follow if their problem is medically the husband's. Couples with female fertility problems may use the egg of a more fertile female and have it fertilized and placed into the wife's uterus for gestation, may contract with a surrogate to carry to term the fertilized egg of a wife without a uterus, or may use artificial insemination with the husband's sperm to fertilize the ova of a surrogate who will carry and deliver the baby. Donor insemination and traditional surrogacy are relatively "low tech" options which have been practiced for a long time. Donor insemination, in fact, has been used in humans since the 19th century. Egg and embryo donation or gestational surrogacy, however, are more complex procedures involving riskier, more invasive, and more expensive assisted reproductive technologies developed during the past twenty years. Some religions have questions about these collaborative reproductive options, and the laws facilitating, supporting or regulating them vary dramatically from state to state and country to country.

There is little data yet available on the long term effects of collaborative reproduction for parents, donors, and children. The professional community continues to disagree amongst themselves about whether donors should be known to those they help and whether children should be advised that they were conceived via collaborative reproduction and offered the opportunity to have information about or even to meet their genetic parents. For the most part, however, we know that the majority of couples who have used collaborative reproduction to achieve parenthood are pleased with the outcome.

As a family member or friend of an infertile couple you should know that a couple considering collaborative options may choose not to tell you about it. Because of society's negative feelings about such options, few couples so far are totally open about having chosen them. Many couples prefer to keep their use of these options entirely confidential, though often this becomes difficult and the couple may take a close friend into their confidence. While such "family secrets" may be difficult to hold, those who have been brought into the decision must be willing to protect and preserve the growing family's privacy at all costs.

A third option for those who cannot give birth to children is adoption. In fact, "You can always adopt," or "Why don't you just adopt? "With all those teenagers pregnant, there must be thousands of healthy babies out there you could adopt!" is the most frequent unsolicited advice couples facing a fertility problem hear. You may be surprised to learn that five percent or less of those who experience an untimely pregnancy plan an adoption these days (and misinformation and misunderstanding on the part of the general public is to a large part responsible for that!—but that's another booklet.) What's more, there are at least forty (some would say as many as 100) couples waiting an average of three to seven years for every baby who does become available for adoption.

The advice to "just adopt" is often followed by an equally disturbing—and wildly inaccurate—comment, "After you adopt, you'll get pregnant! They always do!" Though "everybody" seems to have heard of an exception, for years it has been statistically true—and at the turn of the 21st century it remains so—that fewer than five percent of couples who adopt later spontaneously become pregnant without taking advantage of further intervening medical treatment!

And the final piece of advice potential adopters frequently hear is "If you really wanted a child you'd take one of those kids they advertise in the paper. That's probably God's plan for your life...to take those homeless kids nobody wants." There are 100,000 children waiting for homes in the United States. They are at least of school age, in sibling groups, are emotionally, mentally or physically handicapped or are racially different than the majority of the pool of potential adopters. In general social workers feel that these children with special needs need special parenting skills—skills which are usually developed with experience. Though some of these children will be placed with inexperienced first time parents, many of them will be adopted by families who already have children—people, perhaps, like you? No one should consider adopting a child because they have been incorrectly advised that such is "easy to get" or "all they can get" of "what they should do." This attitude reflects poorly as well on the children who wait, who deserve the dignity of being adopted as a first choice for themselves alone.

A generation ago, in times when unwed pregnancy was frowned upon and birth control less reliable, adoption was a fairly easy, quick, and straightforward option. The picture is different today. The long wait for fewer babies means that couples are being encouraged to explore other adoption options, such as adopting internationally, adopting transracially, adopting a child with special needs, adopting an older child. After using a "should we" tool such as my own *Adopting after Infertility* (Perspectives Press, 1992) infertile people will find a variety of how-to materials to help them in their decision. Books and much more information on forming and parenting families by adoption are available through Adoptive Families of America or their local affiliated parent groups.

Adoption options involve powerful decisionmaking—but it is the couple's decisionmaking, not yours. It is understandable that as family members and friends who know very little about adoption beyond the often inaccurate picture painted in the media, you might initially be uncomfortable with such a choice. But of course you will want to be supportive. You, too, can subscribe to *Adoptive Families* magazine from AFA or to *Roots & Wings* or *Adopted Child* or *Pact Press* newsletters. You can find answers to many of your questions in short booklets such as Pat Holmes' *Supporting an Adoption* and Linda Bothun's *When Friends Ask about Adoption*. Adoption is a wonderful way to build families. Don't allow your ignorance to become a barrier to your participating in your friends' family life.

INFERTILITY'S IMPACT ON OTHER RESOURCES

Though in this booklet we have discussed more thoroughly the emotional impact of a fertility impairment, infertility also takes a physical and financial toll. Testing and treatment involve multiple repetitions of uncomfortable tests. Hormone injections are not just uncomfortable going in, but often create wide mood swings, hot flashes, and other unpleasant side effects, not to mention other physical and emotional discomforts. Nearly all infertility testing and treatment is inconvenient as well as uncomfortable, therefore having an impact on jobs and social life, often in ways which a couple may prefer not to discuss with any but the closest of friends. Testing and treatment are expensive. Few states now mandate coverage, and many employer-provided insurance plans limit its coverage. Microsurgeries and laser surgeries costs thousands of dollars as does each attempt at an assisted reproductive technology.

Financial support for adoption's high expenses is similarly difficult to find. As this booklet is being written, legislation to offer tax credits to those who adopt or deductibility of the many expenses of adopting has not yet passed Congress and been signed into law. It is possible to buy adoption insurance to provide reimbursement for expenses already paid out should an adoption fall through, but premiums are very high and professionals offer mixed opinions about whether the risk is worth it. Though the number is growing, few but the very largest corporate employers yet offer adoption benefit plans to the infertile employees for whom they would have been quite willing to provide childbirth insurance. Many families finance their adoptions by taking out home equity loans, borrowing from credit cards or family members, or working additional jobs for several years.

28

YOU CAN HELP!

Normally, family and friends are the very people who lend support in a time of grief and loss, crisis and confusion, or the joyous chaos of family expansion. The infertile need this same support from their friends and family.

Whatever the outcome of their experience with fertility impairment—whether they become pregnant, choose to adopt, build a family through collaborative reproduction, or decide to embrace a childfree lifestyle—the chances are that an infertile couple will experience great changes as they come through a major passage in their lives.

Infertility is hard work—emotionally, physically, financially. Some ways in which you can support this hard work include:

1. Be ready to listen when one or the other partner or both need to talk. Don't however, offer unsolicited advice unless you are absolutely sure that your advice is factual and needed, and that you are prepared for the possibility that you will be seen as a meddler.

2. Be sensitive. Infertility is an intimate issue of great importance to couples affected by it. Don't joke about it or treat it lightly, and never attempt to negate its importance.

3. Let the couple know that you realize that infertility can be a difficult problem and that you care about them.

4. Be patient. Even without invasive treatment, two week cycles of hope are often followed by several days of crashing despair. When the physical response to medications and the emotional and physical and financial pressures of treatment are factored in, moods may swing even more wildly.

5. Be flexible. At some points couples will find child-centered activities welcome and will want to be involved, but at other times they may need to be allowed to isolate themselves. Don't impose your own behavioral expectations on one who is in crisis.

6. Be realistic. Don't continue to deny the problem or its diagnosis in an attempt to be kind or optimistic. Support your loved one's decision to take a time out from treatment or to stop in entirely.

7. Be supportive. Once you know that the couple has access to expert medical care as it is defined by one of the major infertility consumer support and education organizations, don't second guess or impugn decision making abilities by implying that you know a

"better" doctor and don't raise your personal objections to a chosen treatment or family building alternative.

8. Be truthful. Don't hide your own pregnancy or that of other friends and family members out of "kindness." Instead, respect the infertile couple's need to be told as others are learning of it and try privately to acknowledge that you know that their reactions to pregnancy may be difficult at times and that you want to be understanding about this.

9. Be their advocate yourself. As you hear other family members, co-workers or friends react to an infertile couple or to infertility as portrayed in the media insensitively, take it upon yourself to educate these other "carers" to the pain of infertility.

10. Let the couple know if you are finding it difficult to know what to say rather than saying nothing at all.

11. Remember that because each individual is unique, his or her reaction to infertility will be unique as well. No two couples will necessarily react in the same way, nor will the individual members of a couple experience infertility identically. When, how and if the infertile couple reacts to the stages that have been described here will depend largely upon their own circumstances and personalities. It is not abnormal or unexpected for some reactions to be quite severe. These people are grieving! On the other hand, some individuals may react more stoically.

12. Recommend an infertility support group—RESOLVE, IAAC, INCIID and other groups like them—to those who may not be aware of them. Consider as well, that volunteer-run and donation-supported groups such as these need your financial support as well as the memberships of infertile couples and the professionals who work with them if they are to continue to be able to provide a full range of services.

Somewhere today is an infertile couple luckier than many others. Someone who cares about them—YOU—has chosen to learn more about infertility and what might be done to lighten their load. The fact that you have cared enough to read this booklet speaks well of your potential to be of help to that couple. Remember that neither you nor they are alone.

For more information and for referral to more in depth reading, call Perspectives Press, The Infertility and Adoption Publisher at (317)872-3055 and contact these non-profit organizations:

RESOLVE, Inc. (1310 Broadway, Somerville MA 02144, telephone 617-623-0744) is a U.S. national nonprofit network of 54 chapters offering information, referral, support and advocacy services to infertile people. Dues of $35 annually (includes both national and local chapter membership). Their newsletters, fact sheets and symposia can be indispensable tools. Currently RESOLVE is putting a great deal of effort on a state by state basis into achieving mandated insurance coverage for infertility treatment. They have been successful already in Massachusetts, Maryland, California, and several other states.

INCIID (The International Council on Infertility Information Dissemination) (P.O. Box 6836, Arlington VA 22206, phone 520-544-9548, e-mail HWWK11E@Prodig.com or INCIIDinfo@AOL.com, visit the website: www.inciid.org) A new nonprofit organization dedicated to the exchange of information between fertility experts and those who suffer from infertility. The organization's mission includes expanding the reach of on-line networks to a wider range of infertile consumers, while simultaneously improving the quality and immediacy of available information. INCIID publishes a quarterly newsletter and also conducts an ongoing media campaign to education the general public and garner greater understanding about the emotional, financial, and information struggle facing the infertile. Membership ranges from $25 for consumers to $100 for professionals.)

Infertility Awareness Association of Canada (201-396 Cooper St., Ottawa, Ontario K2P 2H7, CANADA, telephone 613-234-8585, e-mail: iaac@fox.nstn.ca) is a Canadian charitable organization offering assistance, support, and education to those with infertility concerns by issuance of its bilingual publication *Infertility Awareness* five times a year; establishment of chapters to provide grass roots services; a resource centre; information packages; and a network of related services. Services are bilingual (English and French.) Membership is $30 Canadian annually. A complimentary information kit will be sent to interested Canadians upon request.

Ferre Institute (258 Genesee St, Ste 302, Utica, NY 13502, 315-724-4348) is a non-profit organization dedicated to the promotion of quality services in infertility, to the education of professionals the public about infertility and its treatment and to encouragement for research in the psychosocial as well as medical aspects of infertility and reproductive health. Although direct services are offered only in a limited geographic region, their excellent newsletter *FerreFax*, directed primarily at professionals, is available to others.

Stepping Stones Ministry (1804 S Emerson, Denver CO 80210) publishes a monthly newsletter with a Christian focus on the experience of infertility.

The Organization of Parents through Surrogacy (OPTS) (7054 Quito Ct., Camarillo, CA 93012, 805-482-1566) is a national non-profit, volunteer organization with three regional chapters whose purpose is mutual support, networking, and the dissemination of information regarding surrogate parenting, egg donation, sperm donation as well as assisted reproductive technology including IVF and GIFT. OPTS publishes a quarterly newsletter, holds annual meetings, has a telephone support network, and actively lobbies for legislation concerning surrogacy. Membership is $40 annually.

The Alliance for Donor Insemination Families (6067 S Kingston Circle, Englewood, CO 80111-5732) offers support and information for singles and couples considering having a child through donor insemination and parenting support for families already built in this way.

Adoption Council of Canada, P.O. Box 8442, Station T, Ottawa, Ontario K1G 3H8. Phone 613-235-1566. This network collects and disseminates information about adoption throughout Canada, facilitating communication among groups and individuals interested in adoption and promoting understanding of the benefits and challenges of adoption.

Adoptive Families of America, 3333 Hwy 100 North, Minneapolis, MN 55422. Phone 612-537-0316. An excellent source for purchase of books and tapes and of referral to local parent groups, AFA is the largest organization for adoptive families in the world. AFA publishes the 80+page glossy magazine *Adoptive Families* bimonthly. Its Annual Adoption Information and Resources packet lists several hundred agencies nationally and offers consumer advice.

National Council for Adoption, 1930 17th St NW, Washington DC 20009, telephone 202-328-1200. An advocacy organization promoting adoption as a positive family building option. Primarily supported by member agencies, it does also encourage individual memberships from those families who share its conservative stance on open-records and its wary view of open placements. If you have decided to pursue a traditional, confidential, agency adoption, call NCFA for a referral to a member agency.

North American Council on Adoptable Children (NACAC), 970 Raymond Ave. #106, St Paul, MN 55114-1149. Phone 612-644-3036. An advocacy and education resource concerning waiting children, NACAC publishes the periodic newsletter *Adoptalk*, and sponsors each August an enormous, well respected conference on special needs adoption for professionals and parent advocates. This conference rotates through five geographic areas. If you are considering a special needs adoption, call NACAC first for information about local and national resources, parent groups, and adoption exchanges.